Antibodies that Cause and Symptoms

Immune Cells causing Hypothyroidism & Hyperthyroidism

By: James M. Lowrance © 2009

Antibodies that Cause Thyroid Diseases and Symptoms

ABOUT THE AUTHOR:

I am a husband, father, grandfather and lifetime contract salesman, with experience in health writing that began in 2004. I completed theological studies with Liberty University in 1996. I formerly served as editor and forum moderator of Thyroid Health for BellaOnline.com and as a general health writer for Suite101.com, where I received Editor's Choice Awards for my articles on health subjects.

In 2003 I was diagnosed with hypothyroidism; "Hashimoto's thyroiditis" being the cause. This autoimmune form of thyroid disease that causes destruction of the thyroid gland resulted in my also developing "Chronic Fatigue Syndrome", due to a compromised immune system with severe co-morbid "Adrenal Fatigue". I also suffered severe anxiety symptoms, including panic attacks early into the onset of Hashimoto's thyroiditis (Hashitoxicosis). A common heart murmur I was diagnosed with in my teens called "Mitral Valve Prolapse", also worsened in severity of symptoms, with the development of these other health disorders.

TABLE OF CONTENTS:

CHAPTER ONE: Facts about Thyroid Antibodies
CHAPTER TWO: Do Thyroid Antibodies Cause Symptoms Apart From Abnormal Hormone Levels?
CHAPTER THREE: Hereditary Autoimmune Thyroid Disease
CHAPTER FOUR: Epstein-Barr Virus a Cause of Autoimmune Thyroid Disease?
CHAPTER FIVE: Hashimoto's Encephalopathy Rare but Serious
CHAPTER SIX: My Own Experience with Thyroid Antibody Related Symptoms
CHAPTER SEVEN: Autoimmune Hypothyroidism (Hashimoto's) a Cause of Chronic Fatigue Syndrome
CHAPTER EIGHT: Doctors Should Test for Thyroid Antibodies
CHAPTER NINE: At What Point Does Thyroid Autoimmunity Cause Hypothyroidism?
CHAPTER TEN: Medical Research Agrees: Thyroid Autoimmunity Contributes to Symptoms

My eventual receiving of diagnoses was a difficult process with proper diagnostic testing not being ordered by the first doctors I sought treatment from. These types of issues were inspiration for me to become proactive in my own health care and to self-educate myself on these health disorders, which I have done extensively since 2003. I now enjoy sharing this information with other patients experiencing my same health disorders.

CHAPTER ONE

Facts about Thyroid Antibodies

The majority of patients with both hypothyroidism (under-active thyroid) and hyperthyroidism (overactive thyroid) are experiencing autoimmune diseases that cause these conditions. When autoimmune thyroid disease results in hypothyroidism, the terms used in reference to the disease are "Hashimoto's thyroiditis" and "chronic lymphocytic thyroiditis". When the autoimmune disease of the thyroid causes hyperthyroidism, it is referred to as "Grave's Disease" or "toxic diffuse goiter".

Thyroid antibodies attack key proteins within the thyroid gland and in some cases, these will stimulate production of excessive amounts of hormone. These killer cells that are manufactured by the immune system become confused for reasons yet to be fully understood by medical science and they begin to identify thyroid related cells as threats in the body.

As they attack these cells, the thyroid gland becomes damaged over time, resulting in inflammation, enlargement of the gland (goiter) and the resulting thyroid hormone imbalances.

Protein-Enzyme Cell Destroying Antibodies

These antibodies, which are also called "auto-antibodies", enter into thyroid protein-enzymes, causing destruction of them. These targeted proteins are called the "thyroidperoxidase" and the "thyroglobulin". Abbreviations commonly used for these on medical blood lab documents are "TPO ABs" and "TG ABs" or "Anti-TPO" and "Anti-TG".

Once these proteins are destroyed by these antibodies, they are rendered incapable of aiding in the process of converting iodine absorbed by the thyroid gland, into thyroid hormones that regulate the metabolism of all other cells within the body. This is the rate at which the body burns fuels that enter the body, converting them into energy (i.e. food, water and oxygen).

As fewer hormones become available the metabolism can be slowed down (hypothyroidism). These proteins are also part of what keeps thyroid tissue healthy and so as the level of them begins to diminish, thyroid tissue will also begin to die within the gland. As this process occurs, the thyroid gland can become inflamed (thyroiditis) and/or enlarged (goiter).

Thyroid Stimulating Antibodies

These antibodies are also called "Thyroid Stimulating Immunoglobulin" (abbreviated TSI). These type auto-antibodies stimulate excessive release of T3-triiodothyronine and T4-thyroxine from the thyroid gland. They do this by binding to receptors in the blood that normally attach to the Thyroid Stimulating Hormone (TSH) which is another hormone that comes from the pituitary brain-gland and regulates hormone release from the thyroid gland. TSH in-essence is a messenger hormone, telling the thyroid gland how much hormone is needed in the body and it keeps the levels in-balance for proper metabolism via ongoing communication with it.

Antibodies that Cause Thyroid Diseases and Symptoms

Once the TSI antibodies attach to TSH-receptors, the message from them to the thyroid gland mimics the communication of TSH which stimulates an increase in thyroid hormone levels. They are in-essence tricking the thyroid gland into producing more thyroid hormone when it is not needed, resulting in a sped-up metabolism in the body (hyperthyroidism).

Graves' Disease and Hashimoto's Thyroiditis

All three types of antibodies described previously, can be present in both Graves' disease and Hashimoto's thyroiditis. Graves', results in eventual hyperthyroidism in most cases and Hashimoto's results in hypothyroidism. The diseases are differentiated and diagnosed by the balance of auto-antibodies found, by levels of thyroid hormones in the body (imbalances) and by the symptom manifestations caused by the combination of these two factors. The TPO and TG antibodies are typically found in higher titers (lab measurements) in Hashimoto's patients than in Graves' patients, so both diseases cause thyroid gland destruction but at a much slower rate with Graves' disease.

The TSI antibodies that stimulate excessive hormone release from the thyroid gland are found to be high-positive in the vast majority of Graves' patients but are not found to be positive in all Hashimoto's patients and when they are, it is usually in low titers.

If a Hashimoto's patient does have significant levels of TSI, it can cause, intermittent phases of hyperthyroidism, called "Hashitoxicosis" which is a temporary condition, that is usually followed by progressive hypothyroidism.

These facts about antibodies point to how closely related Graves' and Hashimoto's are and may also explain the reason as to why some patients with one disease may transition over to the other in rare cases when a significant change in the balance of auto-antibodies and thyroid hormone levels takes place.

The five subheadings which follow, will review what has been described in the previous subheadings, regarding "thyroid antibodies":

Antibodies that Cause Thyroid Diseases and Symptoms

Thyroid antibodies cause "autoimmune thyroid disease" in patients who develop them.

The immune system normally sends out antibodies, which are killer cells, to eradicate foreign invaders from the body that can make us sick. These invaders include viruses, bacteria and allergens. The purpose of antibodies is to seek these out and destroy them, so as to prevent our bodies from becoming ill. The problem with "thyroid antibodies" is that, like other antibodies that cause autoimmune diseases, they are directed against the thyroid gland as if it is one of these invaders. It is a case of mistaken identity that over time causes damage to the thyroid gland and cell death. Eventually, the antibodies will kill out the thyroid gland completely (hypothyroidism).

Some thyroid antibodies cause hypothyroidism, while others cause hyperthyroidism.

The two main autoimmune diseases caused by thyroid antibodies are "Hashimoto's Disease (thyroiditis), resulting in hypothyroidism, and "Grave's Disease", resulting in hyperthyroidism.

Antibodies that Cause Thyroid Diseases and Symptoms

The types that cause Hashimoto's Disease relentlessly attack the thyroid, until it becomes damaged and unable to function at its original level. Once enough damage has been done to the gland and a significant percent of thyroid cells have been killed, the onset of hypothyroidism occurs. The low level of functioning will usually be mild at first (sub-clinical) and over time will worsen, unless the patient with hypothyroidism receives treatment. The opposite is true of patients with Grave's Disease because in their case, the antibodies directed against the thyroid gland stimulate it to produce excessive amounts of thyroid hormone or a high functioning thyroid gland.

What are the main antibodies tested for in these two types of autoimmune thyroid diseases?

In Hashimoto's Disease, the two main antibodies that cause thyroid gland destruction and resulting hypothyroidism are the anti-Thyroid Peroxidase Antibodies (abbreviated TPO) and the anti-ThyroglobulinAntibodies (abbreviated TG).

Antibodies that Cause Thyroid Diseases and Symptoms

In Grave's Disease, the main antibody that causes stimulation of the thyroid gland to produce too much hormone is called the Thyroid Stimulating Immunoglobulin (abbreviated TSI). The antibodies for both types of diseases are detected by means of blood lab tests.

What are the symptoms that prompt testing for thyroid antibodies that, cause hypothyroidism?

The following symptoms prompt testing for thyroid antibodies that cause an under active thyroid gland:

- increased sensitivity to cold
- constipation
- dry skin
- puffy face
- hoarse voice
- elevated blood cholesterol
- unexplained weight gain
- joint aches, tenderness and stiffness
- muscle pain and weakness
- heavier than normal menstrual periods
- fatigue ...

- enlarged thyroid gland (goiter)
- depression

These symptoms may prompt a doctor to orders tests for the antibodies that cause Hashimoto's thyroiditis, also referred to as "chronic lymphocytic thyroiditis".

What symptoms prompt testing for thyroid antibodies that cause hyperthyroidism (overactive thyroid)?

The following symptoms prompt testing for thyroid antibodies that cause hyperthyroidism.

- sudden weight loss, even if appetite and food intake remains normal or increases
- rapid heartbeat (tachycardia - more than 100 beats a minute)
- irregular heartbeat (arrhythmia/palpitations)
- nervousness, anxiety or anxiety attacks
- irritability
- tremor (fine trembling in your hands and fingers)
- sweating
- changes in menstrual patterns
- increased sensitivity to heat ...

Antibodies that Cause Thyroid Diseases and Symptoms

- changes in bowel patterns (frequent bowel movements)
- enlarged thyroid gland - goiter (swelling at the front-base of the neck)
- fatigue
- muscle weakness
- difficulty sleeping

If one or more of these symptoms are being experienced, this may prompt a doctor to orders tests for the antibodies that cause Grave's Disease, also referred to as "toxic diffuse goiter".

Thyroid diseases can develop at any age but the most common age of onset is between 35 and 40 years of age. It is recommended that adults be tested for thyroid disease at age 35 but they should be tested at any age that symptoms indicating thyroid disease may develop.

Thyroid diseases affect women more commonly than men (from 5 to 8 times more often in females). Pregnancy increases the risk for the onset of thyroid disease and so pregnant women need to have their thyroid function tested as well.

Possible Triggers for Thyroid Autoimmunity

Viruses - Some medical research conclusions have cited the Epstein-Barr virus (EBV) as a possible cause of autoimmune thyroid disease. The research studies state that patients with autoimmune thyroiditis tested positive for blood levels of EBV antigens, significantly more often in the thyroid disease group than in the healthy control group.

While EBV was the virus studied, there are a number of possible viruses that can trigger autoimmune diseases in susceptible individuals. Many of these viruses, especially those in the herpes family, are contracted in early life and carried life-long. It may be that the immune system's failure to fully eradicate the body of these viruses causes it to begin attacking organs or tissues in the body that contain the virus, including the thyroid gland. Some patients, who develop sub-acute thyroiditis (temporary) that is often triggered by respiratory viruses, go on to develop permanent autoimmune thyroiditis.

It may be that these individuals were predisposed to develop thyroid disease once exposed to any number of possible triggers.

Environmental Toxins - Research studies on possible causes of thyroid autoimmunity have also proposed the possibility of environmental toxins as being a common cause for the immune system attacking the thyroid gland. As the body accumulates these toxins, which the body recognizes as allergens or as strong intolerances, the immune system is triggered in trying to control these things that are in-essence acting as poisons in the body. Elevated levels of radioactivity (ionizing radiation), such as may be experienced by those who work at nuclear power facilities or at x-ray imaging labs that are overexposed or not properly protected, can develop autoimmune thyroid diseases. This type of toxin has been well-substantiated as a cause, including studies of children exposed to radiation following the 1986 Chernobyl nuclear power plant accident in Ukraine that caused radioactive fallout. A significant number of children and young adults tested positive for thyroid antibodies in studies conducted 6 to 8 years following the accident.

Other toxins and pollutants that have been studied and that are considered strong possibilities for causing thyroid autoimmunity include toxins found in our water systems, additives and preservatives found in manufactured foods and excessive exposure to fluoride.

Stress - Chronic stress has been studied in relation to many diseases and proposed as a cause for them. This includes inflammatory and autoimmune diseases, types of cancers and immune deficiency illnesses including Chronic Fatigue Syndrome and Fibromyalgia. Many thyroid patients report that they experienced a severe or prolonged period of stress (chronic) just before the onset of their autoimmune thyroid diseases. This association has been better substantiated in patients studied who have Graves' disease, the autoimmune-caused hyperthyroid condition. While less, studies cite stress as a factor in Hashimoto's thyroiditis patients, it would seem obvious that a triggered autoimmune response can result in either condition because all types of thyroid auto-antibodies can be found in both types of thyroid diseases.

Antibodies that Cause Thyroid Diseases and Symptoms

CHAPTER TWO

Do Thyroid Antibodies Cause Symptoms Apart From Abnormal Hormone Levels?

I have corresponded with many fellow autoimmune hypothyroid patients since the year 2003 and have read the testimonies of hundreds of others, in articles and on forums and message boards. What I hear from these patients, is something I have found to be true in my own case as an autoimmune hypothyroid patient (Hashimoto's Disease) and that is the fact that we can continue to experience mild to moderate symptoms, even while on optimal "thyroid hormone replacement medication" treatment. These symptoms can be intermittent or with some patients continual. The more fortunate patients rarely have symptoms while on treatment.

Surveys of thyroid patients on treatment have been conducted, the majority of the patients studied, being on the recommended optimal dose of thyroid hormone replacement medications and many taking natural T-4 and T-3 combination medications.

Antibodies that Cause Thyroid Diseases and Symptoms

The surveys had the respondents to report the effectiveness of their treatments and the results released in these studies, concluded that a majority of patients continued to experience a degree of symptoms.

As I continued to research this subject online, I found research articles by reputable medical research groups, stating that the disease process itself, caused by thyroid antibodies - TPO (thyroid peroxidase antibodies) and the TG (thyroglobulin antibodies), can also be a factor in causing symptoms.

These research articles concluded that elevated levels of these antibodies can cause fibromyalgia type symptoms for example, in persons with only sub-clinical hypothyroidism. Other medical research articles state that autoimmune thyroid disease can also have a degree of systemic (system-wide) effect, so that the immune system response affects not only the thyroid gland but other parts of the body as well.

Antibodies that Cause Thyroid Diseases and Symptoms

Following is a quote from one of those sources:

"However, a responsibility of the mechanisms involved in the autoimmunity rather than a direct action of thyroid hormones seems supported by the evidences that some rheumatic manifestations may occur even in euthyroid patients, or that they are more frequent in hypothyroid patient with autoimmune thyroiditis than in those without this disease."

(PubMed – Title: "Chronic autoimmune thyroiditis and rheumatic manifestations." – Quotes/Reprints are allowed for public education.)

This research article and many others, clearly attribute thyroid antibody levels to symptoms, apart from thyroid hormone levels.

CHAPTER THREE

Hereditary Autoimmune Thyroid Disease

Recently on a Thyroid Health forum I was moderating, a member asked about hereditary autoimmune thyroid disease and what their chances were, as the child of a thyroid disease parent, for eventually experiencing the onset of the disease. Following bellow was my response to that question.

According to Dr. Hossein Gharib, M.D. of the American Association of Clinical Endocrinologists (AACE) and Professor at the Mayo Medical School, "Fifty percent of thyroid disease patients' offspring will inherit the thyroid disease gene."

I actually didn't know that chances for children of thyroid disease parents were at 50% risk until I found that quote from the MD above. I knew it was a high percent risk but 50% was surprising.

That's not great news for children of thyroid disease parents but shows the importance of getting blood tested at any point thyroid type symptoms may arise for both the presence of thyroid antibodies and abnormal thyroid hormone levels and if symptoms don't manifest earlier, to start getting tested at age 35 regardless.

Some reputable thyroid statistics state that between ages 35 and 40 is a common age for the onset of thyroid disease. If you are the child of a parent or parents with thyroid disease, you should educate yourself about thyroid disease symptoms, so that you can recognize when there is a need to be tested, before age 35.

In my opinion, when symptoms arise in someone at risk for developing thyroid disease, they should have not only tests ordered for thyroid function but also the ones to detect "thyroid antibodies". These are the killer cells mentioned earlier that the immune system creates and sends out to attack what it perceives as invaders in the body (i.e. viruses & allergens).

Antibodies that Cause Thyroid Diseases and Symptoms

In the case of autoimmune thyroid disease, it recognizes the thyroid as one of those invaders. These antibodies can cause thyroid disease symptoms in advance of causing eventual thyroid hormone imbalance and is why I believe they are important to have tested in addition to thyroid hormone levels.

To repeat, the thyroid antibodies that should be tested for are the "anti-thyroidperoxidase" (TPO),"anti-thyroglobulin" (TG) and "thyroid stimulating imunnoglobulin" (TSI). Those first two are common findings (found to be positive) in autoimmune hypothyroidism or "Hashimoto's thyroiditis", while that third one is more commonly found in people with autoimmune hyperthyroidism or Grave's Disease, so depending upon the symptoms one is having, they may want only certain ones tested for.

The thyroid function tests, that detect thyroid hormone imbalances in the blood, are the "TSH" (Thyroid Stimulating Hormone), "T-4" (thyroxine) and "T-3" (triiodothyronine) levels. Some Doctors believe the "free" levels of the T-4 and T-3 are best, as opposed to the "total" levels.

Antibodies that Cause Thyroid Diseases and Symptoms

From what I've read in regard to their research on the subject, I happen to agree with them. These are the ones I have tested in follow-up on my own thyroid hormone therapy for hypothyroidism but are also good tests for diagnosing thyroid disorders as well. If only one test is used to evaluate thyroid function, it will usually be the TSH level. This one is the pituitary hormone that accurately reflects how well the thyroid gland is supplying hormone to the body and is sensitive in that it usually detects a change in thyroid function earlier than any other blood test.

Antibodies that Cause Thyroid Diseases and Symptoms

CHAPTER FOUR

Epstein-Barr Virus a Cause of Autoimmune Thyroid Disease?

There is medical research that has been published in regard to the Epstein-Barr Virus (EBV) and its role in causing autoimmune thyroiditis and other autoimmune and neurological diseases. It is also highly associated with contributing to the development of different types of cancer.

I believe that EBV may be the cause of my own Hashimoto's thyroiditis and the resulting hypothyroidism (under-active thyroid) I began to experience at age 39. I suffered a severe case of mononucleosis at approximately 10 years of age that I highly suspect to have negatively affected my immune system.

Thyroid disease, especially the autoimmune type runs in families, in fact children of one parent that has thyroid disease, has a 50% chance of also developing thyroid disease during their lifetime.

As mentioned earlier, Hossein Gharib, M.D., F.A.C.E, president-elect of AACE and Professor of Medicine at the Mayo Medical School states that "Fifty percent of thyroid disease patients' offspring will inherit the thyroid disease gene."

When I personally was diagnosed with thyroid hormone imbalance and later diagnosed with Hashimoto's Autoimmune Thyroiditis, I naturally wondered what caused me to have susceptibility to this disease. I knew that thyroid diseases were experienced far more often in women than in men. My mother however does not have thyroid autoimmunity but did develop age related hypothyroidism, common in women over the age of 60. I also knew my dad does not have thyroid disease or any other type of autoimmune disease. This is what led me to reflect on any childhood diseases that might have triggered the later-life autoimmune thyroid disease I am now experiencing.

When looking back at my childhood, I realized that I developed the severe case of mononucleosis at age 10.

This is the disease caused by EBV (also called "the kissing disease") and after contracting it, the virus remains in your body lifelong. While my siblings (one sister and two brothers), may very well have been exposed to the virus and are now lifelong carriers, they did not experience mono as I did. My mono symptoms were the typical ones, including severely swollen lymph glands in my neck, fever and severe fatigue. In fact, I was taken out of school due to the case of mono, for about six weeks.

My belief is that the virus causing mono in my childhood compromised my immune system and left me vulnerable to developing Hashimoto's thyroiditis as an adult, which also involves the lymphatic system. Another name for Hashimoto's is Chronic Lymphocytic Thyroiditis. I feel it is possible that as the research articles about EBV and autoimmune thyroiditis point out, EBV will cause the immune system over time, to attack tissues in the body that are infiltrated with the virus via antibodies it creates in attempt to eradicate it from the body.

Antibodies that Cause Thyroid Diseases and Symptoms

The immune system is relentless and if it cannot eradicate a virus over time, it may then begin to attack the tissues in the body that contain the virus (autoimmunity). In the case of autoimmune thyroid disease, the immune system creates the TPO, TG and TSI antibodies that replicate to high numbers, to eradicate this mistakenly perceived enemy of the body – the thyroid gland.

When I was rechecked for EBV levels in my blood, shortly following my diagnosis of thyroid disease, I had very high titers of the virus still in my system, as reflected by the antibody levels that correlate with the virus levels. My result on the blood lab test for EBV antibodies (reflecting the level of virus they are attacking) was "218" with normal values being less that "20". My elevations of the virus were more than 10 times the normal range. While I will never be able to prove with certainty that EBV caused my autoimmune thyroid disease, I will always highly suspect that it is indeed the cause in my case.

Antibodies that Cause Thyroid Diseases and Symptoms

CHAPTER FIVE

Hashimoto's Encephalopathy Rare but Serious

There is a neuro-endocrine disorder that causes very serious and potentially life threatening symptoms, called Hashimoto's Encephalopathy (HE). The disorder can occur in patients with Hashimoto'sthyroiditis, who experience a very high elevation of "thyroid antibody" levels. These antibodies, that attack the thyroid gland after recognition of it by the immune system, as a foreign invader, can become highly elevated in these rare cases of HE. At these high elevations they will begin to affect brain and nerve function in the body or the "neurological system". Severe symptoms will result because this system is the body's information and communication center and a disruption from a disease process can cause an array of nerve and brain related symptoms.

Inflammation caused by the antibodies (also called auto-antibodies) spreads to the brain and begins to affect the tissue containing the nerves that control bodily functions and impulses throughout the body.

Antibodies that Cause Thyroid Diseases and Symptoms

The resulting effects are severe neurological symptoms, meaning abnormal responses and manifestations of nervous system dysfunction. These symptoms can include the following.

- psychotic episodes (hallucinations and delusions)
- dementia (mental deterioration)
- neuropathies (abnormal nerve sensations)
- seizures
- coma
- possible death if left untreated.

The antibodies responsible for causing thyroid destruction and inflammation in the thyroid gland but that can rarely also result in HE when highly elevated, are the "TPO" (anti-thyroidperoxidase) and "TG" (anti-thyroglobulin) antibodies. The less common manifestation of chronic lymphocytic thyroiditis, called Hashimoto's Encephalopathy, is more often a result of elevated anti-TPO levels although it can result from elevations of both it and the anti-TG antibodies in some cases.

Antibodies that Cause Thyroid Diseases and Symptoms

Thyroid hormone levels are not usually a factor in this potentially serious neuro-endocrine disorder of thyroid autoimmunity. Some patients in fact have been documented in medical research, to have experienced HE with their thyroid hormone levels falling within normal range and before they were in need of thyroid hormone replacement therapy.

This disorder is a rare but a strong example of the fact that thyroid antibodies have the ability to produce bodily symptoms in some patients, regardless of thyroid hormone levels. I wanted to include information on this rare condition because it demonstrates the direct action thyroid antibodies can exert upon the neurological system within the body.

This would seem to point to the fact that a systemic effect can result from them and this could very possibly be true to lesser degrees as well, such as when patients with thyroid autoimmunity experience disorders of peripheral neuropathy (nerve pain and dysfunction) or dysautonomia (nervous system imbalances), that appear to have no other identifiable cause.

Antibodies that Cause Thyroid Diseases and Symptoms

It would seem that if thyroid antibodies can cause a neurological condition as severe as HE, that they could potentially cause those that are milder or that affect individuals to moderate degrees as well. Only a limited amount of medical research is currently available on this aspect of thyroid autoimmunity.

Treatment for diagnosed cases of HE, is to reduce the inflammation caused by the thyroid antibodies by administering a steroid anti-inflammatory drug to patients who are affected. These drugs, also called corticosteroids or hydrocortisone, mimic the inflammation-reducing properties of our body's own natural anti-inflammatory called "cortisol". A major brand prescribed for acute and severe inflammatory conditions is "Prednisone", a powerful steroid that usually reduces inflammation very effect quickly, with only a relatively short term regimen being necessary to correct cases of HE. Patients, who are treated, usually see a complete reversal of symptoms and will not experience any long term complications from HE, once it has been resolved with treatment.

This is especially true if the condition is diagnosed early into the onset of it.

If a patient with Hashimoto's thyroiditis or their loved ones, notice the onset of sudden and severe neurological symptoms, they should report to their Doctor immediately, to rule out HE as the cause. A delay in treatment for a patient experiencing this very rare disorder could result in severe consequences, such as permanent damage to the central nervous system, brain or spinal cord and in worse case scenarios, coma or death.

CHAPTER SIX

My Own Experience with Thyroid Antibody Related Symptoms

Sometime ago, I had an office visit with an Endocrinologist and I took my LabOne blood test results with me. He found on the results, that my thyroid hormone levels were at optimal range (my free T-3 level was at the top of normal values) but even though I had been on hormone replacement medication for over two years to treat hypothyroidism (via Armour brand -- natural T3/T4 combination), my TG and TPO antibodies were still significantly elevated. My TG ABs, were "537" (normal range <40), so were about 500 points above normal. My TPO ABs, were "120" (normal range <35), so were about 85 points above normal.

My complaint at that time was continuing mild to moderate joint pain, especially in my upper spine and shoulders and moderate, intermittent fatigue. His response to these symptoms I was reporting, was to point out that elevated antibody levels also means that there is resulting "inflammation".

This could cause these rheumatic type symptoms, apart from my normal thyroid hormone levels. I was amazed that other Doctors I had seen previously had never mentioned this possibility and that even the drug manufacturer's websites, did not mention the role of thyroid antibodies, in causing ongoing symptoms, despite proper thyroid hormone replacement therapy for correction of hypothyroidism.

As a result of my unrelieved symptoms, my Endocrinologist prescribed me a short-term round of "corticosteroids" (anti-inflammatory steroid) and told me afterward that I could take occasional over-the-counter anti-inflammatory medications such as Ibuprofen to help with any intermittent symptom-flares. Since that time, my joint pain has diminished to only rare, mild occurrence and I rarely have the need to take an anti-inflammatory for rheumatic (joint and muscle) symptoms but I do still have occasional bouts of mild to moderate fatigue. Occasionally I suffer severe flares of fatigue as well, if I experience chronic stress (lots of added stressors) or if I allow too many stimulants in my diet that I have sensitivities to (i.e. caffeine, chocolate and alcohol).

Antibodies that Cause Thyroid Diseases and Symptoms

I am not sure why more is not being stated in regard to this area regarding the role thyroid antibodies have in causing symptoms because it makes complete sense that highly activated immune system activity, can result in a bodily response manifesting in different degrees of symptoms, depending upon how highly elevated the antibodies are and the resulting inflammation levels. Inflammation from any autoimmune disease process will manifest in symptoms, which means the disease process itself is also what causes illness and this is not restricted only to the hormone imbalances that are involved. Certainly this would be true in cases of autoimmune hypothyroidism as well.

When patients complain to their Doctors about symptoms but their hormone levels are replaced to optimal levels, the Doctor may tell the patient that their symptoms cannot be thyroid disease related because their hormone levels have been corrected. I have heard this scenario related by fellow-patients in my past correspondence with many of them however, when these same patients ask for a retest of their thyroid antibodies levels, and they will often come back highly elevated.

I have heard some patients report TPO levels in the 1,000s which would seem to be a prime candidate for explaining symptom-flares they are experiencing but some Doctors seem to believe the antibody levels are insignificant in relation to symptoms.

It is the opinion of much medical research that has been conducted, that thyroid antibodies do indeed play a direct role in thyroid disease symptoms, apart from thyroid hormone levels and it is my I hope that continued medical research and surveys will be conducted in this area for future treatment considerations.

CHAPTER SEVEN

Autoimmune Hypothyroidism (Hashimoto's) a Cause of Chronic Fatigue Syndrome

While searching for new thyroid disease related information on the web, I came across a medical research article first published in the "Townsend Letter for Doctors and Patents" and re-printed by Dr. Alan R. Gaby M.D.

The article reports a number of findings in regard to patients with "chronic fatigue", stating that a significant percent of them were found in a controlled medical study, to have the type of lymphocytic thyroiditis that causes hypothyroidism (Hashimoto's thyroiditis). The article is titled; "Autoimmune thyroiditis as a cause of chronic fatigue".

The interesting aspect of this report is the fact that these patients were not found to have abnormal (outside of normal values) thyroid hormone levels but despite this fact, they reported that they were suffering symptoms of hypothyroidism.

The autoimmune type of thyroiditis they were suffering from, that was causing the chronic fatigue, was instead diagnosed through a thyroid tissue biopsy called "Fine Needle Aspiration". This is a procedure in which a hypodermic needle is inserted into the thyroid gland and a small sample of gland-tissue is extracted to be analyzed for the presence of diseased thyroid cells.

What is important about this article, is the fact that hypothyroidism does not have to be present, for autoimmune thyroiditis to cause symptoms, such as fatigue, joint pain and muscle weakness. In this case, the research study confirms that the symptom of chronic fatigue is one of those that can potentially be experienced, before thyroid hormone levels become abnormal.

This study is one of many that confirm the development of symptoms from thyroid autoimmunity, in advance of hypothyroidism, that is not yet detectable through blood testing of the hormone levels.

Other medical research articles on the subject of hypothyroid symptoms caused by the thyroid disease process itself, apart from hormone levels, include the development of rheumatic and fibromyalgic type symptoms as mentioned previously.

In addition to my finding these articles and other research for my own articles, through online search, these past several years, I have also corresponded with many thyroid disease patients attesting to having developed hypothyroid symptoms from thyroid autoimmunity, in advance of their thyroid hormone levels becoming abnormal as detected by blood lab test results.

Despite all of the information that is available out there on this subject and reported by the most reputable medical research entities that exist, there are still Doctors treating thyroid disorders, who do not believe symptoms can develop in patients with autoimmune thyroid disease, before thyroid hormone levels fall outside of normal values.

In my own case of being diagnosed with autoimmune thyroid disease - Hashimoto's thyroiditis, also referred to as chronic lymphocytic thyroiditis, I did have abnormal hormone levels on my thyroid panel (i.e. elevated TSH and a low T-3 Uptake), in addition to testing positive for the thyroid antibodies (auto-antibodies) that cause the disease.

My hormone levels were not greatly abnormal but the symptoms I was experiencing, including chronic fatigue were quite severe despite my hypothyroidism not being considered "full-blown" (overt) at the point of my diagnosis.

Even if there were no research articles stating these facts, in my opinion, it is simply common sense to recognize that the disease process itself has symptom-producing potential.

It is after-all autoimmune disease we are talking about and all diseases with autoimmunity as the cause of them, result in inflammation and destruction of tissues in the body that are affected.

Antibodies that Cause Thyroid Diseases and Symptoms

To think that this type disease process only causes symptoms when it affects hormone levels in the body, takes much of the attention away from the seriousness of the disease process that eventually results in the abnormal hormone levels. Chronic fatigue can obviously be one of the early symptoms of an autoimmune disease process in the body, including that which affects the thyroid gland.

Antibodies that Cause Thyroid Diseases and Symptoms

CHAPTER EIGHT

Doctors Should Test for Thyroid Antibodies

Better qualified Endocrinologists, Thyroid Specialists and other types of MDs who treat thyroid disorders, believe in testing for thyroid antibodies.

Sometime ago, I was corresponding with a lady, whose husband was suffering symptoms that matched those listed for thyroid disorder, specifically those of "hyperthyroidism" (i.e. anxiety, insomnia, weight loss, excessive energy, fatigue etc...). Her husband was tested for his TSH and thyroid hormone levels and the results were within the normal ranges however, the man's TSH was on the increase (his result was above 3.5).

According to the new, revised TSH lab standards, set by the AACE (American Association of Clinical Endocrinologists) in the year 2002, this is not a normal TSH level.

The new range suggested by them for revision by blood testing labs is "0.3 to 3.0", with readings above 3.0 are suspect for hypothyroidism, with those falling below 0.3 being suggestive of hyperthyroidism. In my discussion with this woman, who was seeking help on behalf of her husband, I told her that her husband's TSH would also merit tests that detect the presence of "thyroid antibodies".

Following was my reply:

"A TSH of 3.58 is not as normal as some Doctors would have you believe. The AACE which is the organization that sets the standard for thyroid testing and treatment, released a new, revised TSH range in late 2002, having "3.0" as the cut off for high-normal TSH.

Here's a quote from the AACE:

"Now the AACE encourages physicians to consider treatment for patients who test outside the boundaries of a narrower margin based on a target TSH level of 0.3 to 3.0." (The AACE)

The National Institutes of Health website actually states that a person testing with a TSH of above 2.0, should be monitored closely for development of thyroid disease.

Here is a quote from the NIH:

"Some people with a TSH value over 2.0 mIU/L, who have no signs or symptoms suggestive of an under-active thyroid, may develop hypothyroidism sometime in the future."
(NIH/NLM - MedLinePlus.com, reprints allowed for public education.)

My suggestion to you is to find a qualified thyroid-treating Doctor and to have your husband tested for the possibility of being positive for thyroid antibodies.

These can reveal the presence of thyroid disease, in patients with normal-ish hormone levels. The tests are for the "TPO, TG and TSI" antibodies and a positive reading on one or more of these indicates thyroid autoimmunity is occurring.

People with developing autoimmune hypothyroidism (Hashimoto's thyroiditis) for example, can have elevated antibody levels that cause symptoms, even with hormones being within normal-range. Patients with Hashimoto's thyroiditis (most common cause of hypothyroidism in industrialized countries), can experience a period of hyperthyroidism, before the onset of hypothyroidism begins and progresses and the term for this temporary condition is "Hashitoxicosis".

Here is a quote from a page on the WiKi website:

"Hashitoxicosis is an autoimmune thyroid disorder, in which individuals with autoimmune hypothyroidism, usually Hashimoto's thyroiditis (HT), experience intermittent or sporadic periods where they also have symptoms of hyperthyroidism." (Graves' Disease and Hyperthyroidism - WikiWebsite Page)

Amazingly, some Doctors will argue these points, despite the fact that the most reputable medical sources available are stating them.

Antibodies that Cause Thyroid Diseases and Symptoms

Some Doctors believe and state that antibody testing is not necessary unless hormone levels fall outside of the normal reference ranges but the fact is that autoimmune thyroid disease is usually present long before it affects the hormone levels, in causing them to become imbalanced.

This would be my suggestion; to get him tested for "thyroid antibodies". It may confirm or rule out thyroid disease but will be difficult to move on to other possible causes of his symptoms, if they are not tested for.

Some Doctors jump to snap-diagnoses of emotional problems, such as anxiety and depression, before ordering more complete blood evaluation for patients with both mental and physical symptoms and in my opinion, this is a disservice to them. I believe people with multi-symptom complaints, should not only be tested for thyroid hormone levels and thyroid antibodies but they should also have a complete blood count (CBC) and glucose levels (A1C) tests, to check for diabetes and other blood disorders."

(End of my reply.)

CHAPTER NINE

At What Point Does Thyroid Autoimmunity Cause Hypothyroidism?

The e-mail response below, I made to a woman writing to me about being diagnosed with thyroid autoimmunity. In other words, she was found to have immune cells attacking her thyroid gland, also called "thyroid antibodies". I went into some detail about these antibodies that cause thyroid disease and in how they correlate with the development of hypothyroidism.

My E-Mail Response:

"As you said in your e-mail, the "1120" (highly elevated) lab result you quoted was the TPO antibody or "anti-thyroidperoxidase", which is positive more commonly in people with autoimmune thyroid disease than is the anti-thyroglobulin (TG), when thyroid disease is caused by the immune system (thyroid autoimmunity).

Antibodies that Cause Thyroid Diseases and Symptoms

The immune system sends out these auto-antibodies to attack the thyroid gland because it has for some reason recognized it as an enemy in the body, as it normally would with germs, bacteria, fungus or allergens.

In some patients both antibodies can be highly positive but even if only the TPO is positive, this already indicates autoimmune thyroid disease. Thyroid autoimmunity as it is also called is the most common cause of hypothyroidism in the US and other industrialized nations. The specific name for this inflammatory condition, is "Hashimoto's thyroiditis".

I don't have your full story but if you are already being treated, you are just finding out the cause (autoimmune) of your hypothyroidism or at least the cause of your hypothyroid type symptoms. If you're not yet being treated, you likely will be soon but Doctors vary in what they consider to be the stage at which to treat a patient with thyroid autoimmunity, which is also showing signs of progressing into a hypothyroid state.

Some factors involved in treatment decisions include the degree of symptoms being experienced and whether or not a goiter (thyroid enlargement) is present.

The "TSH" (Thyroid Stimulating Hormone), the pituitary hormone that monitors and stimulates thyroid hormone production will usually become abnormal first (it elevates early with hypothyroidism) and afterward the thyroid hormones "T-3 and/or T-4" will begin to fall below the normal range as well. The TSH does the opposite and begins to elevate when a person's thyroid begins to fail. It is the hormone that stimulates the thyroid, so when it rises, that means it is having, to send an abnormally high amount to keep the thyroid working at proper level."

(End of my reply.)

CHAPTER TEN

Medical Research Agrees: Thyroid Autoimmunity Contributes to Symptoms

In this chapter, I will be commenting on a recently published medical research article about autoimmune thyroid disease. I would first like to make comments in regard to symptoms some patients with autoimmune hypothyroidism caused by Hashimoto's thyroiditis, experience that many medical Doctors may tell them, is not thyroid disease related.

Autoimmune hypothyroid patients will report to their Doctors, that they suffer systemic (system-wide or body-wide) joint and muscle aches. Patients will report experiencing neurological symptoms (nervous system) and sicca symptoms (areas of bodily dryness). These types of symptoms will be experienced by these patients even with their hypothyroidism being treated by hormone replacement therapy, to correct the low thyroid hormone levels.

Doctors will many times respond to patients, by telling them that these type symptoms are not thyroid disease related but are rather emotionally based or possibly even imagined (psychosomatic).

When further testing is then done and no further causes for their symptoms can be found, doctors may then resort to the psychosomatic or emotional diagnosis. There is however more medical research being published, that clearly states that the autoimmune process itself that causes hypothyroidism, is an additional cause of symptoms, apart from abnormal hormone levels. In other words, the thyroid autoimmunity or disease process itself contributes to symptoms and may continue to do so in some patients, even after low thyroid hormone levels from hypothyroidism, are corrected.

With my continual searching on the internet for new information about autoimmune thyroid disease, I occasionally run across medical research articles that stand out on particular subjects.

In the case of the one I wish to comment on following, several technology publishing groups, have published conclusions by a medical research body, specifically "The Department of Pathophysiology, Medical School, National University of Athens, Greece", that looks at the subject of the "systemic manifestations of autoimmune thyroid disease". It makes some statements that are in my opinion, very important for those in the medical community to make note of, in regard to thyroid patients.

The research article is titled "Systemic Autoimmune Manifestations: When Should Underlying Thyroid Autoimmunity be Considered?" Within the abstract of this article that is indexed on websites and search engines for public view, it states that this research group has reported clinical and laboratory data suggesting that "thyroid autoimmunity" could be involved in the symptomology of some patients who experience systemic/rheumatic symptom manifestations.

The abstract also states that symptoms in these categories, such as musculoskeletal complaints and neurological manifestations, are not uncommon in patients with autoimmune thyroid disease, which affects approximately 10% of the general population. In my opinion, this abstract/article which I personally located on the IngentaConnect.com website makes some extremely important observations and statements in regard to the role of thyroid autoimmunity in causing the symptoms of autoimmune thyroid disease.

With so much medical research and patient testimonials offered on the subject of the role of thyroid antibodies in both the thyroid disease process and its symptoms, doctors and patients alike should become better informed on this subject, especially as it relates to the effectiveness of hypothyroid treatment success.

(END)